Skin Care

Homemade All-Natural Makeup and Beauty Products

Beauty Clinic Josephine

derived from various sources. Please consult a licensed professional before attempting any techniques outlined in this book.

By reading this document, the reader agrees that under no circumstances is the author responsible for any losses, direct or indirect, which are incurred as a result of the use of information contained within this document, including, but not limited to, — errors, omissions, or inaccuracies.

Table of the contents:

What is natural and is it still the best? 8

Making your own cosmetics and beauty products 9

To start..14

Understanding the skin 14

Skin types 16

Three-step skincare routine 18

Supplies...21

Is our water clean? 35

Buy essential oils..35

Moisturizing ingredients...37

Emollients 38

Occlusive..38

Humectants 39

Emulsifiers and detergents 40

Emulsifiers 40

Emulsifying wax 41

Use emulsifying wax 41

Alternatives to emulsifying wax 41

Detergents / surfactants..42

Preservatives...45

Parabens 46

Appropriate preservatives 47

Antioxidants 48

Storage and shelf life of homemade products 48

Creams, gels and lotions 49

Lip balms, butters and ointments 50

Oils for face and body 51

Bath bombs and salts 52

Tips, tricks, and the basics 52

For the face 61

Hydrating neroli spritzer 66

Regenerating serum for the skin 68

The oils 69

Green clay cleansing mask 70

Hydrating vitamin mask 73

Apricot face scrub 74

Lip balms 77

Soft butters 77

Facial cleansers 78

Face scrubs 81

Face masks 83

Facial toners and astringents 86

Face moisturizers 90

Other face care products 93

Full face makeup 94

To make loose powdered makeup solid 95

Liquid foundation 103

Body care 110

Soaps 111

Bath soaks 113

Body scrub 114

Body moisturizer 115

Hair care 116

Conclusion 121

My answer is always the same - just because it's natural, it doesn't make it safe, and just because it's man-made, it doesn't make it dangerous. Most of the ingredients used in skin care are processed in one way or another to make them usable. The essential oils are steam distilled and the oils are machine pressed. Look for botanical ingredients that have the least amount of processing and are as close to their natural source as possible, and don't be afraid to use a small amount of safe synthetics to make some products more functional.

The term "green" means different things to each of us depending on our lifestyle. For some, this simply means recycling and reusing the carrier bags; for others, it means composting, growing organic vegetables and cycling everywhere. When creating skin care products, decide your expectations for their performance and the tradeoffs you are willing to make. For some, emulsifiers and preservatives may be out of the question, limiting the types of products you can do. For others, you might be willing to compromise 5-6%

greenness for a more sophisticated product - every sight is good, too.

Organic certification has become a major focus for eco-care brands, but I wonder if we've lost sight of some real issues here. Should we be shipping ingredients halfway around the world just because they're organic and avoid the good local producers because they don't have organic certification? Should we buy organic products rather than non-certified fair trade, or should we support fair trade cooperatives regardless of their organic status? You will have to make up your own mind about what is important to you, and it will be different for everyone.

Hope you find the recipes both fun to make and fabulous to use. Feel free to experiment and if you find a great variation let me know!

Making your Own Cosmetics and Beauty Products

With the vast numbers of cosmetics and beauty products on the market, many people wonder why anyone would want to make their own. Then again, people are also becoming more health conscious and thus understand the point of using products that you are very familiar with (because you made them!). There are many brands out there that tout natural ingredients and wondrous benefits, but there is always a question about how much of that is marketing and how much of it is actually true. Finding the right product can also be difficult if you have certain sensitivities, allergies, and health concerns. Of course, you can personalize your own products however you'd like. There are a multitude of reasons to make your own bath and beauty products.

When it comes to labeling beauty products, there is often some discrepancy between what the label says and what the product actually consists of and does. Even brands that claim they are made with all natural ingredients and are safe for all skin types may use fillers, ingredients that can irritate certain skin types, and even chemicals. (By chemicals, we are referring to synthetic ingredients; obviously, everything is a chemical in some sense.) Even the "natural" ingredients may be ultra-refined and processed versions of the raw ingredient. Though this is not necessarily bad, it can mean that the key properties and benefits of the ingredient have been altered, diluted, or even cooked out altogether. There is currently no comprehensive regulation of many bath and beauty products, making mislabeling and misrepresentation a much more common issue than people would think.

Second only to food and beverages in allergenic potential, external body products are an issue for anyone who has sensitive, oily or dry skin; allergies and sensitivities to certain ingredients; or other relevant health issues. One example is tree nut allergies: People with this type of allergy are unable to use products containing coconut, shea, hazel nut, almond, pecan, walnut, cashew, pistachio, or Brazil nuts. Many natural products use coconut oil and/or shea butter, and some even use almond oil. Alcohol is used in a lot of commercially made body products, and this can be drying to the skin and even painful to people with rashes, wounds, and sensitive skin conditions.

Not only can you make sure your homemade makeup, soaps, and moisturizers are safe for you and your skin, you can also tailor them to your wants and needs. The shades of color, glossy or matte, dark or light —you can make it how you want it. If you haven't been able to find that perfect shade of green, you can use micas and pigments and slowly work out a formula that creates your dream color. You can find natural essential oils or fragrance oils of almost any scent imaginable to make your lotions, soaps, and scented sprays smell exactly as strong or light as you please. For most of the recipes in this book, there is a vast amount of tinkering you can do to make the final product exactly what you want.

When purchasing the ingredients for homemade bath and beauty products, you will often be surprised at how much you can make with the amount you bought. Although some things, such as essential oils, may seem expensive, a little goes a long way. You will end up with a much larger quantity for a lot less money than if you'd bought a store brand. There are also options like eBay, Etsy, and wholesale sites to get bulk amounts more cheaply. And many of the ingredients may very well be things you already keep in your home: cocoa powder, cinnamon, coffee, coconut oil, olive oil, and so on. Many of the tools are basic kitchen utensils; you just have to clean and sanitize them first. You'll be surprised at how much you can make with few to no extra purchases.

With homemade products, you have control of both quantity and quality. You can make a small amount of a certain shade of eye shadow or scented lotion, or you can make enough to give as holiday gifts. Many oils, fragrances, and colorants are interchangeable, meaning that you can buy whatever type fits your budget and preference. If you aren't set on the base oil being almond or hemp, you can use less-expensive olive oil.

As you can see, there really are quite a few reasons to start making your own bath, body, and beauty products. Time may be an issue for some, and the convenience of store-bought products is undeniable, but for the most part making your own is very much a "pro" rather than a "con." You may even enjoy it so much that you make a business out of it, and if nothing else, the joy of using something you made yourself, or giving it to someone you care about, is extremely satisfying. No one will know your product as well as you, and you will know everything that went into making your ideal cream, soap, makeup, or facial mask. (Not to mention that makeup made with things like cocoa powder and cinnamon smells absolutely delicious!)

This book should be a good starting point, a stepping stone in your journey to become your own alchemist of beauty.

I know the temptation is to skip this chapter and jump straight to creating the recipes that follow, but please take a moment to read these pages. Here you will find good advice on the materials and the different types of ingredients used in recipes, as well as essential information on the use of preservatives and the shelf life of your creations. There are skin care and beauty guidelines from the inside out as well, and once you get the basics down you can create your own variations of my recipes.

Understanding the skin

The dermis

This layer is quite resistant with a lot of elasticity since it is mainly composed of connective tissue composed of collagen and elastin. As we age, the collagen fibers, which help bind water to the skin and give it strength, decrease and wrinkles begin to develop. If the skin is stretched too much, as in obesity and pregnancy, the elastin fibers can rupture, resulting in stretch marks. The dermis also contains hair follicles, sweat glands, sebaceous glands, blood and lymphatic vessels, and sensory nerve endings.

The sebaceous glands are located near the hair follicles and are found in all parts of the body except the palms of the hands and the soles of the feet. They secrete sebum - a mixture of oils and fats - in order to keep the skin lubricated and to provide waterproof protection. Sebum also acts as a bactericidal and antifungal agent to prevent germs from invading the skin. The sebaceous activity is regulated by the male sex hormone androgen, which is present in both men and women and increases at the onset of puberty; this is why oily skin and acne are more common at this age, especially in adolescents.

The epidermis

The outermost layer of the skin itself is made up of several layers. The basal layer, at the bottom, also known as the stratum germinativum, is where new cells are created. During their 40-

day cycle, cells gradually move from the basal layer to the stratum corneum at the surface, where they are shed through a process called "desquamation". New cells will then take their place and the cycle will start again.

The basal layer is also the site of melanocytes, which are responsible for the pigmentation of the skin - the production of melanin. Melanin production is actually your body's defense mechanism against the harmful rays of the sun.

SKIN TYPES

ORDINARY

If you are lucky enough to have neither particularly dry nor oily skin, then it is could be classified as normal and should just be kept clean and hydrated with simple, light cleansing lotions. Many skins fall into what is called the category of combinations. Combination skin is where the "T-zone" of the forehead, nose, and chin is slightly oilier than the cheeks. Cheeks aren't necessarily dry, but most of us produce more oil in the center of the face. Don't be afraid to treat each area with different products if necessary. If you always seem to have a shiny nose, don't use moisturizer as it obviously produces a lot of oil on its own.

OILY

Although more prone to clogged pores and blemishes than dry skin, oily skin has the advantage of looking younger for longer. However, they can also be prone to dehydration and sensitivity, so take this into account when choosing your treatment. Avoid strongly occlusive ingredients, as they can cause rashes, and include plenty of water-based humectants instead. Choose lighter oils, such as thistle, rice bran, and jojoba, avoiding coconut oil and butters like cocoa and shea, as they can block pores.

DRY

Skin with underproduction of sebum needs extra help to stay beautiful smooth and supple. Adding richer oils and butters to your products not only helps trap water in the skin, but also smoothes out rough edges of epidermal cells, resulting in a smoother appearance. Gently cleanse and use protective moisturizers in winter as well as in an air-conditioned area the environment, as this tends to make dehydrated skin worse.

The three steps to healthy skin are keeping it clean, protecting it from dehydration and the elements, and dealing with any problems that arise.

1 keep it clean

Since sebum is sticky, it attracts dirt and debris from the environment and should be removed with regular cleaning to prevent pores from clogging. You can't stop sebum production or close pores, and neither should you want to because they both perform vital functions. For some people, using soap or detergent-based cleansers on the face disrupts the acidic mantle of the skin and makes it dehydrated and uncomfortable. The answer here is to try a cleansing lotion, oil or balm instead. Since I have oily skin and like to wash my face with water, I use either a cleansing balm or an oil removed with a washcloth or cheesecloth (muslin). For years I have used foaming facial cleansers (because I was nervous about using something oily), but I always felt they irritated my skin. I now use the Basic Manuka Honey Cleansing Balm (see p. 31), and my skin feels much better for it.

Personally, I don't advocate constant exfoliation with facial scrubs, and I think the skin does a good job on its own if treated properly. With that said, using a washcloth or cheesecloth (muslin) twice a day will remove excess dead cells, which probably has something to do with it. I would only use a scrub very occasionally if my skin looked a bit dull.

2 Protect it from dehydration and the elements

There are two things you can do to help your skin look and feel better: keep it moist and protect it from trans epidermal water loss (TEWL). Trans-epidermal water loss simply means that the water in your skin evaporates when subjected.

to the elements, leaving it dehydrated. Ingredients in skin care products such as humectants have the ability to draw more moisture from the air to the skin's surface, but they cannot hold it. This is where ingredients like emollients and occlusives come in, as they help slow down the evaporation process while keeping the top layer of cells soft and supple. Sometimes we want to create a protective barrier, but if the barrier is too thick it can block pores and cause blemishes, so choose your ingredients carefully for your particular skin type.

3 Solve problems

Facial skin problems can be very debilitating. Personally, I believe that an issue on your skin indicates that something is out of balance on a deeper level. Much of conventional medicine and skin care focuses on correcting symptoms and what you can see rather than looking for the cause. We can all be guilty of this too, as our main concern is getting rid of the offending stain quickly. While it can work in the short term, if the original cause is left untreated, the defect, in one form or another, will always reappear.

Tackling skin problems is all about understanding what's normal for you. For example, I know that my diet, my physical activity, and my stress levels can take their toll on my skin. If they are in balance, my skin is beautiful; otherwise my skin looks terrible and suffers from all kinds of weird pimples. The occasional monthly breakouts are normal for me, but nothing more than that means I have to put my life back on track. I visit an herbalist or homeopath for more problematic skin issues because I don't want to be given antibiotics or steroid cream just to make the problem go away.

1. Equipment

It is best to use different equipment for making your makeup, bath, and body products than you use for cooking. This keeps irritating cooking ingredients and ingredients that will spoil quickly from ending up in your products, and it also keeps product ingredients that aren't safe to ingest out of your food. If you are tight on funds, it is okay to use your kitchen cookware, but you should make sure to thoroughly clean and sanitize it before and after making personal care products.

<u>Coffee or Spice Grinder or a Mortar and Pestle</u> – Even if you are able to get dry ingredients in powdered form, a fine grinder is great for blending powdered makeup.

Mortar and Pestle – Great for grinding ingredients into fine powder

<u>Containers for products</u> – Whether you use clean baby food jars and old makeup containers or buy jars/pots/bottles, you will need something to put your liquid and powdered finished products in. Check the resources section for a list of places that you can purchase both specialty and low-cost containers.

<u>Double Broiler</u> – This set-up consists of a metal or glass pot or bowl that sits above a pot of boiling water. Since this method doesn't use direct heat, you can melt ingredients without the risk of burning them. If you do not have a double boiler, you can use a microwave-safe glass dish and heat the ingredients up using short "bursts" from the microwave (usually 15–30 second intervals).

<u>Funnels</u> – If you are making any liquid products (liquid soap, lotion, toners, etc.), you will need a funnel to get them into containers.

<u>Kitchen Scale</u> – These scales measure much lower weights than most scales. Some come with a container on top, others have a flat top, but they can all measure the smaller quantities you will be using in making your own products. You'll need one because some ingredients are given in weights rather than volumes due to how they are sold and stored. (As an example, cocoa butter is often in irregular chunks which couldn't be measured accurately with spoons or cups.)

<u>Measuring Cup</u> – I actually use Pyrex measuring cups for mixing as well as measuring. Why? Well, Pyrex is very durable, heat resistant, clear glass so you can see if anything has settled or separated, and has the perfect spout for pouring. The smooth glass also makes it really easy to clean up.

<u>Measuring Spoons</u> – If possible, getting a one-milliliter measuring spoon (like the tiny feeding spoons in a Sea Monkey kit) is wonderful. In any event, you will need measuring spoons from the smallest size you can find up to a tablespoon.

<u>Mixing Bowls</u> – Mixing bowls should have smooth sides (not textured or with lines) and be resistant to heat if you are making anything requiring melting or heating ingredients. It's best if they have a pour spout on the lip in case you need to pour anything into bottles or jars.

<u>Pipettes</u> – These come in disposable plastic or as glass with a rubber end. Pipettes are good for getting drops of essential oil or vitamin E oil.

<u>Sifter</u> – A sifter is necessary for breaking up clumps in fine powdered ingredients and to make sure the ingredients are properly combined. Cocoa powder, for instance, likes to clump up, and you have to use a sifter to break up the clumps so that you can mix your base powder with the cocoa powder thoroughly enough. There are two types of sifters: an ice-cream scoop shaped one with a screen "spoon" and a handle that sends a curved piece of metal or plastic along the screened bowl of the spoon, and a cup shaped one with the screen on the bottom and a flat piece of metal or plastic that moves when you squeeze the handle, pushing the powders apart and through the small holes in the screen.

<u>Stick Blender</u> – Also called wand blenders, these are great for mixing wet ingredients in bath and body product making. You can stick it in any bowl or measuring cup, swirl it gently as it blends, and get the proper blend of ingredients with easy clean-up. A standard blender can be used, but they are harder to clean, often too big for the quantities you'll be making, and more costly.

2. Ingredients

Obviously you only need the ingredients for the recipes you wish to try; this is just an overview of the ingredients most commonly used in natural bath and body product and makeup creation. For our purposes, everything should be cosmetic grade or food grade.)

<u>Activated Charcoal Powder</u> – This powder is used as a black colorant. It's made from hardwoods or coconut shells that have been exposed to high heat. The resulting charcoal is then ground into a powder.

<u>Aloe Vera Gel</u> – Light green to clear liquid extracted from the leaves of an aloe vera plant. This liquid is great for skin irritations and to help moisturize dry skin.

<u>Allspice (powdered)</u> – An herb often used in cooking but also useful as a brown colorant when in powdered form.

<u>Apricot Kernels (ground)</u> – The dried and ground seed/pit is used as an exfoliant in scrubs and soaps.

<u>Arrowroot Powder</u> – The separated and dried starch of various tropical plants. This is used as a base in many natural cosmetic products and is less likely to cause negative skin reactions than commercial mineral makeups.

<u>Beeswax</u> – This can be bought in chunks, pellets, wafers, and even bars. The smaller the form you can get it in, the better. When you get beeswax in large chunks or bars, you have to shave off portions or melt it down to cool it in smaller bits to use in your recipes. To cut or shave it, you can use a cheese shredder or a knife (aiming away from you as you cut off small strips), but you'll find that you waste a lot of it this way.

Unrefined Beeswax

Beeswax can also be bought raw (yellow) or filtered and deodorized (white). The choice is really up to you. Although the yellow color won't show up in the quantities used in body products, some people prefer it to the processed kind. The raw beeswax still has remnants of honey and small amounts of minerals that are beneficial and worth keeping.

Beetroot Powder – Beets are dried and powdered to get this pink to mauve/maroon colorant.

Blueberry Seeds – Dried seeds are used as an exfoliant in scrubs and soaps.

Castile Soap – Sold in liquid or solid form, castile soap is made with natural oils and lye. It's great to use on its own or as a base in home-crafted soaps.

Cinnamon (powdered) – Finely powdered cinnamon is used as a "warm" brown colorant. Cinnamon can be irritating to some skin types.

Clay (Kaolin, Bentonite, Rose) – Clays are beneficial in face masks and powdered makeup. Different types are good for different reasons. Kaolin is white, ultra-fine, and very absorbent. Rose is pink clay that's great for sensitive skin. Bentonite is a grayish-white clay made from volcanic ash; it is used to help with skin conditions and speed up healing processes.

Cocoa Butter – Cocoa butter is a solid oil that comes from the cocoa bean. Often it has a creamy color and a chocolate scent. You can buy deodorized versions that lack the smell and color, but these will have been heated, which reduces the beneficial properties. Cocoa butter is a fantastic moisturizer and skin rejuvenator. It can help reduce scars and stretch marks when used regularly and helps skin stay healthy. This solid oil melts on contact with the skin and absorbs fairly well. If you are allergic to chocolate or caffeine, cocoa butter may not be a safe option.

Cocoa Powder – Cocoa powder is what is left after the cocoa bean has been dried, the cocoa butter removed, and the remaining matter pulverized. It can be used both as a brown colorant and for energizing and rejuvenating soaps and scrubs. Do not use if you are allergic to chocolate or caffeine.

Coconut Oil – Coconut oil is extracted from the pulp of the white coconut meat. Raw coconut oil may have a light scent. Like other oils, it can be bought refined and odorless, but the amount of beneficial minerals is reduced during the heating process. Coconut oil is a great skin moisturizer and can help with irritation. It is also a wonderful makeup remover! Although the likelihood of a reaction is low, you may wish to avoid coconut oil if you are allergic to tree nuts.

Coffee (finely ground) – Regular coffee, unflavored, and ground up finely (not powdered, just finely ground) is often used in invigorating scrubs. You can also use espresso. Do not use if you are allergic to coffee or caffeine.

Cornstarch – A fine, white powder extracted from corn. It is used as a thickener and as a base in powders. Cornstarch is very absorbent.

<u>Distilled Water</u> – Water from the tap or an outside source can contain bacteria that could cause your products to spoil or become unsafe. If you decide to use water that is not distilled, make sure to boil it ahead of time to kill any lingering bacteria.

<u>Essential Oils</u> – Essential oils (unlike fragrance oils) are extracted directly from the plant, herb, flower, tree, root, or fruit. There are many types of essential oils with aromatherapy properties and even minor healing properties (for stings, dry skin, burns, etc.). Essential oils are best when "cold-pressed" and not heat extracted. This helps retain their vital nutrients and properties. Essential oils are only to be used in very small amounts, as they can be irritating to the skin when in concentrated form.

These oils are often diluted when being applied directly to the skin or burned in an infuser. Be careful using them, and always test a product containing essential oils on a small area of skin first, to make sure there is no reaction. The most commonly used oils in natural body products are lavender, chamomile, flower scents, and tea tree oil (one of the few safe in concentrated form, though it is still irritating to the eyes).

Glycerin (vegetable) – Vegetable glycerin is made from plant-based oils, most often coconut or soy. It is usually food grade. Glycerin is used as a carrier for many other oils and a blender for non-oil liquids with oils.

Honey – Honey is a natural antimicrobial and antibiotic with an extremely long shelf life. It enhances the body's own healing processes, moisturizes the skin, and even acts as a natural preservative.

Iron Oxides – Iron oxides are used as colorants. They are pigments extracted from minerals. Iron oxides are most commonly black, red, yellow, and brown.

Melt and Pour Soap – Soap base made with vegetable glycerin and lye, which may also include aloe, goat's milk, honey, oatmeal, and other ingredients. It is prepared in a way such that it can be easily melted and altered with other ingredients for simple home-crafted soaps.

Mica – Micas are pearlescent pigments extracted from minerals. They are used for shiny and sparkly colorants in body products.

<u>Nutmeg (powdered)</u> – Dried and powdered nutmeg is used as a goldenbrown colorant.

<u>Oil (Olive, Sunflower, Grape Seed, Hemp)</u> – Oil is necessary for body products such as lotions and creams. Olive oil is the most common choice, but this heavier oil has a tendency to go rancid faster than others if not properly stored. Most oils are interchangeable, though, and which one you use will depend on preference more than any other factor. In general, whichever is cheapest or easiest to obtain will work fine in the recipes in this book.

<u>Palm Oil</u> – Although it's been getting a rather bad reputation on social media, there's nothing intrinsically wrong with palm oil. It's extracted from a variety of palm trees, and many providers of this solid oil list detailed information about where they get their oil from. Palm oil is useful as it does not cause problems for people with tree nut allergies like coconut oil and shea butter can, and provides similar benefits.

<u>Pigments</u> – Iron oxides and micas are pigments, but there are also powdered colorants made from flowers, plants, and even fruits and vegetables. Unnatural colors often contain chemicals, so check to see what the source is for the pigments you choose.

There is a vast variety of colorants made from natural things that can provide a good spectrum of color options without making your makeup less natural and healthy.

<u>Rose Water</u> –Rose water is a hydrosol (water infused with plant matter) that can be used in place of distilled water in beauty recipes to gain the benefits of rose oil for clear and clean skin. It can be bought, or made as follows: Rinse fresh rose petals. Place in a pot and cover with distilled water about ½ inch above the petals. Lightly boil for about half an hour, let cool, and strain. For the longest shelf life, store in a sealed container in the refrigerator.

<u>Rubbing Alcohol (or Vodka)</u> – Alcohol is a common ingredient in commercially sold cosmetics, but it can dry out the skin. However, I do use alcohol for a few things when making natural products at home: sterilizing equipment, as a fast evaporating liquid when compressing powders, and in perfumes (because it evaporates on warm skin, leaving behind only the scent instead of an oily residue).

<u>Salt</u> – Used as an exfoliant and in bath soaks, scrubs, soaps, salts, and similar products. Salt isn't great for dry skin unless a moisturizer is used afterward. Salt can also be painful in soaks if you have any open wounds.

Shea Butter – This is a solid oil that comes from the shea nut. As with other oils, it has a creamy color and a strong scent in its raw state but can be purchased deodorized and refined, but containing less nutrients. Not as hard as cocoa butter, shea butter is still firm and melts on contact with the skin, meaning that it's easily absorbed. It is used for moisturizing skin and helping with skin conditions, much like cocoa butter. Some people combine the two or prefer one over the other, but their properties are really very similar. If you have an allergy to tree nuts, do not use shea butter.

Silicone spatulas and molds – Silicone spatulas (the ones with the rubbery ends instead of hard plastic) and silicone molds are great for making bath and body products as they are super easy to clean with soap and warm water. The silicone spatulas are fantastic for scraping clean a bowl or cup so as to waste as little as possible. Wood absorbs oils and is difficult to properly clean, while hard plastic spatulas and molds are less efficient, difficult to unmold from, and break more easily.

<u>Spirulina (powdered)</u> – Dried and powdered algae used as a dark green colorant.

<u>Strawberry Seeds</u> – Dried seeds used as an exfoliant in scrubs and soaps.

<u>Sugar</u> – Sugar is often used in scrubs and in-home body waxes. You can use raw sugar or refined sugar; the choice is up to you. Sugar is abrasive enough to exfoliate the skin, but won't dry it out like salt can.

<u>Titanium Dioxide</u> – Titanium dioxide is a processed mineral used as a white colorant and to help provide sunscreen-like protection in homemade products.

<u>Vanilla Extract</u> – Used to brown products and add a sweet fragrance.

<u>Vitamin E (oil or capsules)</u> – Vitamin E comes in bottles of oil or in capsules. Vitamin E oil is fantastic for skin protection, moisturizing, reducing scars and stretch marks, and minor healing improvements. Often a recipe will call for so many drops or so many capsules. To use the capsule, poke a small hole in it with a pin or needle and squeeze the gel exterior to extract the oil into your mixture.

<u>Witch Hazel (liquid)</u> – Witch hazel is made from the bark and leaves of the witch hazel tree. This liquid is great to help clean skin and stop skin irritations, and as a base for astringents and toners.

<u>Zinc Oxide</u> – Zinc oxide is a mineral used to add sun protection to body products.

Is Our Water Clean?

Although it is clean enough to drink, it is not clean enough to be used in beauty products unless a preservative is added. Use distilled water or spring water. If you only have tap water, it should be filtered and boiled.

Buy essential oils

Of all the ingredients you'll use in your homemade beauty products.

Essential oils can be the most expensive, so it pays to do your research before spending any money. Rather than spending hours scouring the web for the often confusing and contradictory information, buy a good book and follow its advice, including important security considerations you should be aware of. when you are dealing with essential oils.

Tinctures, Glycerols, and C02 Extracts These latter types of extracts are too difficult for most of us to make at home and are best purchased from a reliable herbal supplier.

Tinctures are made by steeping herbs for a fairly long time in a mixture of alcohol and water. They are primarily sold by herbalists for internal use, but many skin care companies add them to their products. Due to their alcohol content, tinctures may not be desirable in products for sensitive skin, as they can have a fairly drying effect. The solution is to use glycerol (glycerin extract) instead.

The advantage of a glycerol is that the herb is macerated in glycerin, which is both water soluble and a humectant. This means that it is suitable for both water-based products and those containing an emulsifier, such as creams and lotions. Since glycerin is not soluble in oil on its own, use oil macerates in products that contain only oils and waxes (or an emulsifier).

CO2 extracts are the result of a fairly new (and expensive) process known as supercritical CO2 extraction, which is used to create herbal and plant extracts for use in the cosmetic, food industries. and herbal. The plant material is rinsed with carbon dioxide under high pressure, which acts as a solvent to release the volatile components of the plant. Due to the lower temperatures involved, it is used to extract essential oils from plants without using chemical solvents when steam distillation is not possible. It is also used to make herbal extracts, which can be added to your products.

The CO 2 vanilla extract is particularly useful because the vanilla absolute is not soluble in oil and is difficult to incorporate into products, while the CO 2 extract works perfectly.

Moisturizing ingredients

There are three types of moisturizing ingredients used in creams or lotions emollients, occlusive, and humectants - and the challenge is to combine them for the best effect. Understanding their basic functions and how they work together will make it much easier to create your own recipes from scratch or edit any of the recipes in this book.

Emollients

These help improve the appearance of the skin by softening, smoothing and increasing its suppleness. For my recipes, these will be natural vegetable oils and butters, ranging from very light and easily absorbable oils, like thistle, to richer and heavier butters, like coconut and shea. Some oils, like borage and hemp, are high in essential fatty acids and vitamins but are not particularly emollient and will feel quite dry on their own. For this reason, it is good to include a few different oils in each recipe, to improve the performance and feel of the skin. For each recipe, I've included information on the oils so you get a good idea of what works for different skin types.

Occlusive

These reduce trans-epidermal water loss (TEWL) by creating an impermeable barrier on the skin, and they work best when applied to slightly damp skin. Some emollients, such as cocoa butter, have occlusive properties, as well as waxes such as beeswax, which make them great for making barrier products to protect the skin from the elements. Some occlusives are quite comedogenic (aggravating acne) and should be avoided on skin prone to pimples or acne. Many skin care experts are against occlusive ingredients because they are believed to prevent the skin from breathing; however, for some areas, like the lips, hands, and feet, they are good at creating a protective barrier on dry, cracked skin.

Humectants

Glycerin, honey, and hyaluronic acid are all humectants. Although they are still moisturizers, humectants work in a different way from other moisturizers by drawing water to the skin to keep cells plump and hydrated. Once the water has been drawn to the skin, you need additional ingredients, such as emollients and occlusors, to hold it in.

Products like lip balms, body butters, and skincare balms are relatively easy to make, and the right ingredients can usually be obtained these days to make them 100% organic. If, however, you want to make a more sophisticated cream or lotion, you'll need to use both an emulsifier to blend the oil and water-based ingredients, and a preservative to keep them from going out.

Emulsifiers

In simplistic terms, the role of an emulsifier is to make oil soluble ingredients adhere to water soluble ingredients in the same way you would add egg yolk to oil and vinegar when making making mayonnaise. It works because the egg yolk contains lecithin, which has emulsifying properties.

If you are making a lotion or cream, you will also need to add a thickener to get the right texture, as an emulsifier alone will only create a milky liquid. Some natural emulsifiers that you can buy have thickening properties, but in most cases you will need to add an additional ingredient.

Emulsifying wax

The most commonly found and easiest to use emulsifier for home use is emulsifying wax, which is an umbrella term for a number of different formulas. Some types of emulsifying wax contain thickeners and some do not. If you are not sure, ask your supplier or just try a recipe. If it's too thin and watery, you may need to use a separate thickener.

Use emulsifying wax

I have found that using emulsifying wax at 25% of the total fat content with no butters or thickeners creates a thick, but still pourable lotion. If you want to make a thicker cream, add a little more emulsifying wax or add cetyl alcohol to the recipe.

Alternatives to emulsifying wax

In addition to emulsifying wax, there are many emulsifiers used in the food industry that are available to the home craftsman, and you might prefer to use them instead - or at least experiment with them. I have found that for most of the recipes in this book, swapping 5% emulsifying wax with 5% glyceryl monostearate plus 2-3% cetyl alcohol works very well, although it does provide some texture. slightly thicker. I've also included a recipe suitable for oily skin (see p.46) using a new emulsifier (and probably the greenest on the market today) — Olivem 1000 - which seems to work very well in light lotions..

Ingredient search

If you are concerned about an ingredient, do your own independent research as new studies are being done and new information is being discovered every day. When you read "studies show," try to find the studies and read them yourself.

Detergents / surfactants

If you want to make your own bath and shower gels, you will need to familiarize yourself with a group of ingredients known interchangeably as surfactants / detergents. Most of the homemade recipe books do not cover this type of recipe as these ingredients are considered to be villains that should be avoided at all costs. While I agree that the area of detergents and surfactants is a minefield when it comes to being green and eco-friendly, I also think it's important to know why the ingredients are rated good or bad. Even if you decide not to make the detergent recipes in this book, I hope you have a better understanding of the ingredients used and empowered to make more informed choices when buying over the counter.

There are plenty of naturally occurring detergents on the market that are based on sugars, coconut or palm oil, but don't be fooled by the illusion that they would occur without intensive chemical treatment. Just because something is naturally derived doesn't automatically make it skin-friendly and biodegradable, so always check with the vendor you're purchasing from or search for INCI names online if you're unsure. (As languages vary across the world, a common language has been devised for labeling requirements, meaning that each ingredient has an INCI name, pronounced "ink"). It is possible that some ingredients that we now consider "good" and approved by organic certification bodies could be further criticized - this is the nature of the industry.

To be as environmentally friendly and environmentally friendly as possible, avoid detergents that are:

Petrochemicals Derived Obviously, as a non-renewable source, any petroleum derivative should be avoided if you are looking to be greener.

Harsh on the Skin Since the whole purpose of a detergent is to dissolve the oil and allow it to be rinsed off with water, many detergents can be quite abrasive to the skin and in some cases irritating.

Non-biodegradable If a detergent is not biodegradable, it will remain in the water after being rinsed in our sewers, damaging fish and flora.

So what is a surfactant?

Without getting too technical, a surfactant is a substance that affects the surface tension of water (a surfactant). It consists of molecules with hydrophilic (which love water) heads and hydrophobic (which hate water) or lipophilic (which love oil) tails. Put simply and in the context of a shower gel, dirt and oils in the skin stick to the lipophilic end and are flushed down the drain through the hydrophilic end. Easy!

The detergents I have used in my recipes are those commonly used by natural skin care companies which are also readily available to the home craftsman. There are a lot more, so if you want more information, take a look at the resources section at the end of the book (p.143) where I've included the best links I've found for further reading.

Preservatives

Along with detergents and emulsifiers, preservatives are the cosmetic ingredients that always concern those of us who want a greener, more natural skincare product. Having the word "preservative free" on the label is probably the holy grail of natural cosmetics, but that is really not possible for most commercial products because they are produced in huge quantities long before they are sold. This is when making your own cosmetics has definite advantages, as you can make small amounts of them that require fewer or no preservatives.

Any product made with water needs a preservative to keep it from going out and becoming both unpleasant and potentially harmful. If you want to avoid preservatives altogether, your only choice is either to make products that do not contain water, or to prepare a very small amount and store them in the refrigerator, using no more than a week or two (see p.26 for more information) on the manufacture of products without preservatives). Products containing botanical extracts, such as herbal infusions and floral waters, have a much higher risk of contamination with yeasts, fungi and waterborne bacteria, and therefore require additional preservatives.

Preservatives are under constant scrutiny from regulators because by their very nature (killing microorganisms) they can harm us too. It is quite common to use two or even three preservatives in a mixture to ensure that all contaminants are eradicated. For example, some are good yeast inhibitors but are not effective against waterborne bacteria. Other factors that determine the effectiveness of a preservative are the pH of the product and its compatibility with other ingredients, such as emulsifiers and detergents.

Parabens

They are the most controversial conservatives. At one time, they were used by most skin care companies because they were both effective and unlikely to cause allergic reactions. However, many natural skin care brands have started reformulating the products, due to a study (which has since been discredited) that linked the parabens in deodorant to breast cancer. Currently, the American Cancer Society says there is no scientific evidence that parabens increase the risk of breast cancer, and the FDA considers them to be safe for use in cosmetics. However, just because there is no current evidence that there are no long term effects, and you will have to decide for yourself whether you are willing to take the risk or not. It should be noted that anything rinsed from the body, such as shower gel, is less likely to be absorbed into the skin than a leave-in product, such as cream or lotion.

Appropriate preservatives

The other main issues with preservatives are their propensity to cause allergic reactions, as well as safety issues such as some release formaldehyde. On p.142, I've listed those available in small quantities to make your own products at home. Although unnatural, they are the best available today. Check out the ones listed and check out the online forums as there are many artisans trying out different formulations and have some great experiences to share.

Many publications mistakenly refer to ingredients such as vitamin E and rosemary seed extract as "preservatives" when in fact they are antioxidants. So what's the difference?

Oxidation occurs when the product comes into contact with air and begins to decompose or go rancid. Just as an apple turns brown if the skin has been cut, it is a natural rotting process. No outside factors or contaminants should be involved, it's just something that happens naturally when molecules react with oxygen in the air. Keeping products in an airless package and using antioxidants, such as vitamin E and rosemary seeds, will slow this process.

Since products made from oils and waxes are not prone to microbial contamination, they will only need an antioxidant, such as vitamin E, rather than a preservative.

Storage and shelf life of homemade products

All of the recipes in this book include a preservative or antioxidant, if needed, to extend the shelf life and freshness of the products, in some cases up to a year or more. However, I'm sure many of you will want to make fresh, natural products with minimal chemical additives. This section therefore gives guidelines on storage and shelf life without preservatives.

A good place to start for extending the shelf life of your homemade products is to create a super clean work environment, using equipment specifically reserved for making products you don't use for cooking. I like to use metal and glass because they are easy to clean and less likely to harbor bacteria. Before you start working, wipe down your equipment and counters with isopropyl alcohol or rubbing alcohol, available at most drugstores. You can decant a small amount in a spray bottle to spray the surfaces and wipe them down with paper towels; make sure the bottle is clearly labeled and kept in a safe place, as alcohol is flammable.

Creams, gels and lotions

The key thing to remember when determining the shelf life of a product is whether water has been added in any form (this includes bottled spring water and hydrosols, or floral waters). If this is the case, the finished product should be stored in the refrigerator and will not last more than a week or two at most;

treat it like a dairy product. The shelf life of a cream or lotion will also depend on its packaging: if it is in a jar that opens every day and has your fingers soaked in it, its shelf life will be shorter than a product kept in a bottle with a pump dispenser, which not only prevents fingers from entering, but also prevents air from being drawn into the bottle. You can buy an airless pump distributor packaging from some ingredient suppliers.

Adding herbal ingredients to your products (especially herbal teas) will also reduce the shelf life as they are a great growth medium for bacteria. If you notice any mold on the top, thinning or separation of the product, strange smells or a change in color, throw it out!

Lip balms, butters and ointments

They are products with no added water and simply made from oils, butters and waxes. Balm-type products do not produce mold and fungus, but they will eventually turn rancid over time, depending on the oils used. If you notice that a product is developing mold, it means that water has entered it. So, in the future, make sure your bottles and jars are completely dry before use.

To assess the shelf life of your product, check the expiration dates of the ingredients used and choose the one with the shortest shelf life to be on the safe side. Some oils last a year or two, but some, like rose hips and borage, will go rancid within a few months if an antioxidant like vitamin E is not added at the time of pressing. It is a good idea to buy these oils with an antioxidant already added, if possible. The action of heating the oils and butters during the manufacturing process of your products, as well as the addition of 0.5 to 1% vitamin E oil (which all the recipes in this book contain), will be enough to Extend the life of your body butters, ointments and balms up to 1 to 2 years, as long as you are using oils whose expiration date is met.

Oils for face and body

These are similar in nature to balms and butters in that they will not mold but will oxidize over time and become rancid. Since you don't heat them, they won't last as long as the balms, but they should last about a year with 0.5–1% added vitamin E (depending on the shelf life of the base oils used). All reputable suppliers must include an expiration date on the ingredients; if they don't, contact them to verify. If you make your own macerated oils with fresh plant materials, they should last 6 to 12 months, but don't forget to add vitamin E as an antioxidant.

Bath bombs and salts

Bath bombs and salts will not go away, but should be kept in moisture resistant containers to keep them at their best. If the bath bombs get wet they will start to dissolve and the salts can sometimes get a bit solid, so it is best to keep them in airtight kitchen containers.

Tips, Tricks, and the Basics

Although all of the recipes in this book have been successfully created, there is a bit of trial and error to learning how to make beauty products at home. Some ingredients have certain quirky properties or can be fickle. Many of the recipes are not difficult at all, but if you aren't used to working with certain ingredients, you may get frustrated with them.

It's okay if it doesn't turn out right the first time. You can try to salvage it or scrap it and move on. Your best bet is to make the smallest batch possible the first time, so that you have an idea of how it will come together and what the end product will be.

Always write down what you are doing. Especially if you are one to stray from specific recipe instructions! Keep a notebook and jot down every ingredient you add, the amount you used, and what you did after you added it. This can help you when you want to recreate something, or if you want to look back and see where something could be changed.

Properly store all ingredients and final products. Anything that uses an oil, like olive oil, has the potential to turn rancid. This isn't to say you need to put it in the refrigerator, but you should try not to leave oil-based products in hot and/or humid environments. If it's been a while since you made it and something smells "odd" or "off" to you, you can spot-check it on your arm, but you may want to dispose of it. Sanitizing containers, working in a clean environment, and using distilled water can also help preserve your products.

Always clean your work area and tools before and after making anything. This prevents cross-contamination between food and beauty products, and will also help prevent any bacteria or debris from causing problems with your food or your products.

Double Boiler versus Microwave Some ingredients must be heated up or melted to use them in a recipe. When you heat these ingredients (oils, waxes, butters, etc.), you cannot have them touching the heat source, as that would cause them to burn. High heat can also result in fires with certain oils. Therefore, you should use either the double boiler method or the microwave method.

For a double boiler, fill one pot a third to half full with water, enough to reach at least a quarter inch up the bowl or pot you put on the top. The bowl or pot must be able to sit on top of the pot of water safely. For bowls, you will have to use glass or metal. Be very careful, as these bowls will get extremely hot and they do not have handles. As the water boils in the pot underneath, the ingredients in the bowl or pot on top will melt.

For the microwave, use a microwave-safe bowl or measuring cup. Heat in 15–30 second "blasts," stirring after each one to prevent hot spots and burning. You do not want to overheat any ingredients; they only need to be hot enough to melt and combine.

Essential Oils (EOs) versus Fragrance Oils (FOs) Many recipes, forums, and websites refer to these oils as EOs and FOs. EOs are essential oils, or oils extracted directly from the plant, fruit or vegetable. They are sold in concentrated form and often need to be diluted. A little goes a long way. They have many therapeutic uses and are a very common ingredient in natural products. FOs are fragrance oils that are often a combination of essential oils, extracts, and other oils to make a specific scent. Many FOs have a vanilla or citrus extract base. Vanilla extract based oils can cause some browning as the final product ages. It is only a cosmetic change, though, and does not affect the product.

Speaking of EOs and FOs, there are some other terms and abbreviations you might want to familiarize yourself with before you seek more information on making products. There are actually a lot of them, but here are some of the most frequently used:

- OO – Olive Oil
- VOO – Virgin Olive Oil
- EVOO – Extra Virgin Olive Oil
- CP Soap – Cold Press Soap (a soap-making process that uses lye)
- HP Soap – Hot Press Soap (a soap-making process that uses high heat and lye)
- MP Soap – Melt and Pour Soap (soap made from a pre-made base of vegetable glycerin that does not need lye and is merely melted, mixed with other ingredients, poured into molds, and ready to go after it is cooled)
- CO – Coconut Oil
- ACV – Apple Cider Vinegar

Raw versus Refined Oils, butters, and waxes come in a few forms. Raw is usually cold processed, i.e., not extracted with heat, and contains the highest amount of nutrients and minerals. Raw forms are often colored, scented, and may even have a slight texture because they haven't been processed.

Refined has been heated, and the scent and color is a lot less noticeable, but it may also be a little less rich in minerals and nutrients. Ultra-refined or deodorized is usually clear or white and unscented. This form is sometimes bleached and heated to high temperatures. This is the form most commercial brands use. Ultra-refined and deodorized butters, oils and waxes have very little of the original benefits remaining and are simply used for the fat content required in some recipes (such as soap and lotion).

Liquid and solid oils and butters Different oils and butters become solid and liquid at different temperatures. Liquid oils are rarely solid unless chilled or frozen, as they have very low melting points (this includes most cooking oils – olive oil, safflower oil, grape seed, etc.). Solid oils and butters have higher melting points and can be solid at room temperature (shea butter, palm oil). Cocoa butter is classed with the solid oils but is sometimes also referred to as a "brittle butter" because of its harder form.

Know what you want to make before you buy ingredients. Many ingredients are cheaper in bulk, but you will use only small quantities of the most expensive ingredients. Know what you plan on making before you order ingredients. This also applies to making sure you get the right pigments for makeup, the right ingredients for your skin type for soaps, and so on. Commercial products are filled with preservatives and will last practically forever; natural products aren't and won't (although there are some natural preservatives you can use to help extend the shelf life of your products). If you make a large quantity of something you do not plan to use much of, it may spoil or become rancid before you can use it all. Plan ahead.

Know your ingredients. Make sure you always test your product on a small spot on your forearm. Wait a bit and see if there is any reaction, especially if you're using any new ingredients. Check the ingredients you use and take note of any safety warnings. Just because something is natural does not necessarily mean it is harmless.

Coconut oil is your face's friend. After making makeup, you are going to want to try it on. Again, the forearm or wrist is the best place for this. First, check and make sure there are no reactions. Second, see if the color, shimmer, and shade is what you wanted and how it will look against your complexion. Once you have makeup on, though, you will eventually want to remove it. If you are experimenting with different shades and colors, you will be removing a lot. Coconut oil dabbed on a napkin or soft cloth can wipe makeup off with no irritation and no need to scrub. It also helps moisturize the skin. Use only a small bit; it is oil, after all. Massage it in and then wipe it off.

Natural means natural. Crazy and outrageous colors of makeup that are completely natural are hard to come by. You have to accept that natural makeup will have a more limited color palette. The same goes for shelf life, due to the lack of preservatives to keep the natural oils from going bad. Another thing many people do not realize is that natural soap and cleansers do not bubble and foam nearly as much as commercial brands. Detergents are added to make those soaps foam up; it's not a natural occurrence from the ingredients. Your homemade soaps may still bubble a bit, and coconut oil based soaps and fizzy balls can have some foaming properties, but it won't be a thick lather like store-bought brands.

Save makeup containers. Empty eye shadow and blush compacts, lip balm and gloss pots and tubes, and mascara tubes and wands can be washed in hot soapy water and reused to put your own products in.

Parts and ratios Some recipes tell you to use a ratio such as 1 part oil and 2 parts water. When you see this, just take the amount you use for the 1 part and multiply it by the number of parts specified for the other ingredient. Example: The recipe calls for 1 part coconut oil to 2 parts aloe vera and you want to make it with ½ cup of coconut oil. Multiply ½ × 2 = 1 cup of aloe vera. If you look up other recipes online, you will see this type of measurement a lot. If there isn't a specific measurement for the ingredients, use the smallest "part" first and then multiply how much of that you used times the parts required for other ingredients. (This is usually used in recipes that aren't written to make a specific amount of product, and you won't find it in this book as often as you would online.)

Liquid makeup can go bad, even the store-bought kind. Whether it is mascara, foundation, lipstick, or a bottle of some fancy wrinkle serum, pay attention to how it looks and smells when you purchase it. Although many people are turning away from chemical based makeups, those do have preservatives in them to delay issues with bacteria and rancidity. Natural makeup often does not have this protection. Honey, Vitamin

E, and polysorbate (a preservative made from vegetable oil) are sometimes used, but there is still a risk of the product going bad. The last thing you want to do is put rancid or bacteria-riddled makeup near your eyes and mouth, so be sure to store all natural makeup in a cool, dry place. Some recipes in this book actually require refrigeration to keep the products good for the longest amount of time. Be cautious and use your instincts; if you think something is bad, do not use it.

For the face

Facial care products are very simple to make with good quality natural ingredients and can be just as effective as store bought ones. Most of us are much more careful and picky about the products we use on our face than the products we use on the rest of the body - and rightly so, because facial skin is much thinner and more prone to hair loss. tenderness and irritation. For this reason, I tend to avoid using a lot of different essential oils in my facial products and sometimes leave them unscented or just add a few drops of essential oil to mask the strong oil smells. basic. This chapter includes recipes for everyday cleansers, toners, and moisturizers, as well as special treats, such as face masks, eye serums, and lip balms.

Macadamia & Jojoba cleansing oil

I'm sure you're wondering why I called this "Macadamia & Jojoba" when the biggest ingredient is, in fact, castor oil. Well the simple fact is that "castor oil" doesn't sound very appealing, and this is an example of why skin care products are often named after their more exotic ingredients rather. than their biggest ingredient. However, the manufacturers are not trying to defraud us, as such, just to seduce us!

Despite its unglamorous name, castor oil is an extremely effective cleanser: it attracts dirt and grime on itself and is very slow to absorb into the skin. It is quite viscous, so it must be mixed with other oils to allow it to spread more easily; choose other slow absorbing oils like macadamia, apricot or avocado. I have also included jojoba in this cleansing oil because it is suitable for all skin types and does not block pores.

If you intend to use the cleanser to remove eye makeup, do not add essential oils as they can irritate your eyes.

Ingredients

2 tbsp (30ml) macadamia oil 40ml castor oil

5 teaspoons (25 ml) jojoba oil

1 teaspoon (5 ml) of vitamin E oil

10 drops of essential oil (optional): Normal / dry skin: chamomile, sandalwood, geranium, rose Oily skin: tea tree, lavender, lemon, cypress, juniper

Equipment

small glass or metal jug airtight metal spoon

100 ml (3½fl oz) glass bottle with pump dispenser

1 Add the oils, one at a time, to the glass bowl.

2 Add essential oils, if necessary, and mix well.

3 Carefully pour into the glass bottle and close it.

USE

Massage into skin to loosen makeup or dirt. Remove the cleanser with a damp cotton ball followed by a quick wipe with floral water or toner. You can also remove it with a washcloth soaked in water or a damp muslin cloth.

Lavender and Witch Hazel Deodorant

Skin fresheners, or toners, are something we've all been encouraged to use in the past as part of a cleansing, toning, and moisturizing routine, and though they seem to have fallen out of favor. , I've included a few different options for you. here. If you take a look at the ingredient list of most good quality natural toners, they are mostly made up of either water with the addition of herbal extracts or floral waters. Floral waters, or hydrosols, are the by-product of the steam distillation of plant materials during the production of essential oils. For this reason, it is quite easy to get a wide variety of different floral waters, which can be used on their own as skin fresheners or mixed with other water soluble ingredients. Hydrosols go away fairly quickly unless a preservative is added, so you will usually need to use them within six months.

Witch hazel bark is distilled not for its essential oil but for the sole purpose of producing distilled witch hazel, which has a variety of uses in and of itself. This hydrosol is ideal for oily skin because it is slightly astringent, and it makes an effective eye lollipop in summer if you suffer from hay fever.

Ingredients

2 teaspoons (10 ml) of witch hazel

85 ml of lavender water

½ teaspoon (2.5 ml) of yarrow tincture

½ teaspoon (2.5 ml) of vegetable glycerin

Equipment

100 ml (3½ fl. Oz.) Spray bottle

1 Measure and simply pour all four ingredients into the spray bottle.

2 Screw on the lid firmly and shake well to mix.

USE

Always dilute witch hazel with spring water if using it around the eyes, as it is quite strong, and use a maximum of 2 teaspoons (10 ml) to 3 fl oz (90 ml) The water.

Hydrating Neroli Spritzer

This hydrating spritzer is in the same spirit as a toner, but it is less astringent and more suitable for normal, dry or sensitive skin. You can add any ingredient to a water-based spritzer like this, but the ones that are not water soluble, such as essential oils, will float upward, so you will still need to shake the spritzer before use.

Orange blossom water is the by-product of distilling orange blossoms to make neroli essential oil. Neroli and orange blossom water are good for sensitive, aging skin and people with broken capillaries.

Aloe vera concentrate is also soothing and can be added to any type of toner or refreshment for its anti-inflammatory properties.

I used vegetable glycerin in this recipe for its humectant properties, but you could replace it with hyaluronic acid, which would be even better.

Ingredients

2 teaspoons (10 ml)

aloe vera

85 ml orange blossom water

teaspoon (2.5 ml) of calendula tincture

½ teaspoon (2.5 ml) of vegetable glycerin

Equipment

100 ml (3½ fl. Oz.) Spray bottle

Hyaluronic acid

Hyaluronic acid is used in commercial anti-aging skincare products and is naturally present in the skin. It can absorb several times its own weight in water and is responsible for giving the skin its roundness and rosy appearance. This naturally decreases with age, especially after 50 years, which contributes to the formation of fine lines and wrinkles.

Note that hyaluronic acid in commercial skin care can come from rooster combs, but it is also available as a by-product of bio fermentation, which is the version generally available to the home artisan online. (but check to make sure).

1 Simply add all the ingredients to the spray bottle.

2 Screw on the lid firmly and shake well to mix.

The oils used in this blend may be a little new to you, but they are all readily available online. If you want to make your own anti aging skincare products that actually have some effect, it's worth looking into these specialty oils, which are all packed with vitamins and antioxidants. Take a close look at Latin names and compare them to the ingredients listed on your favorite products: I'm sure you'll be surprised at the similarities.

Note that all of these oils can also be incorporated into any lotions you make, so don't just save them for the serum.

Ingredients:

4 teaspoons (20 ml) kiwi seed oil

2 teaspoons (10 ml) rice bran oil

1 teaspoon (5 ml) pumpkin seed oil

1 teaspoon (5 ml) of argan oil

1 teaspoon (5 ml) borage oil

1 teaspoon (5 ml) of vitamin E oil

5 drops of essential oil (optional)

Equipment

small glass pitcher or airtight metal spoon beaker
50 ml (1½ fl. oz.) glass bottle with dropper

The oils

Rice bran oil has been used for centuries by Japanese women
for their skin. Nourishing properties, and it is used to
protect against premature aging.

Kiwi seed oil is absorbed into the skin very quickly and
does not leave a greasy residue, making it perfect for all skin
types.

Argan oil has recently gained popularity as an anti-aging
skin oil. It comes from the argan tree, which grows in certain
regions of Morocco. It is very rich in vitamin E and linoleic
acid.

Pumpkin seed oil has a fairly high zinc content as well as
vitamins A, C and E, as well as omega-3 and omega-6 essential
fatty acids. It is used in skin and body care products for its
lifting effect on the skin.

1 Add the oils one at a time to the glass bowl.

2 Add the essential oil, if necessary, and mix well.

3 Carefully pour the mixture into the glass bottle.

USE

Apply a few drops to freshly cleansed skin, alone or under a moisturizer for an extra boost.

Green clay cleansing mask

When I do masks for myself at home this tends to be a thing to use in the moment. Clay masks dry very quickly if you only use water or an infusion of herbs, so they really need to be prepared in a small, fresh amount for each use. This recipe is for a single use mask and can be tailored to suit any skin type by changing the essential oils, infusion, and type of clay used - just keep the same amounts and you'll be fine.

This mask is for those times when one cleanser is just not enough. Lavender and juniper oils are both antiseptic and decongestant; aloe vera will help soothe inflamed or irritated skin. Green clay is full of minerals and will help remove dirt and toxins from your pores as well as soothe the skin; It is suitable for all skin types.

Set aside 20 minutes to relax while your mask works on your skin. The best way to do this is to soak in a hot tub, which will also help open your pores.

2 teaspoons (10 ml) of lavender water or herbal infusion ½ teaspoon (2.5 ml) of aloe vera concentrate 1 teaspoon (5 ml) of green clay 1 drop of 'juniper essential oil 1 drop of lavender essential oil

Equipment

small glass bowl or egg cup

Since it is such a small amount, it is very difficult to weigh the ingredients accurately on most kitchen scales.
You will find it much easier to use measuring spoons instead.

1 Add the lavender water or herbal tea and aloe vera to the small bowl.

2 Sprinkle green clay over the liquid and stir well, using the end of ateaspoon.

3 If the mixture is still too wet, add more clay; if it is too dry, add morelavender water until you have a nice thick paste that is easy to spread on your skin.

4 Add the essential oils, stirring well.

USE

Run a hot tub and wrap your hair in a towel or shower cap. Prepare your mask and apply to freshly cleansed skin, avoiding eyes and lips; if you having too much for your face, apply the rest to your neck and chest. Relax in the bath for 15 to 20 minutes. If the mask starts to feel too tight as it dries, moisten it lightly with water. To remove the mask, hand dip a clean washcloth in warm water and place it on your face to moisten the mask. Remove the mask with the damp cloth, being careful not to rub and rinse the cloth several times. To finish, rinse your face one last time with clean water or use the rest of your infusion or a little flower water as a finishing rinse.

Hydrating vitamin mask

I love using honey in skin care products for its moisturizing and skin lightening properties. Homemade masks (especially those that use clay or food ingredients) are best made in single-use amounts because they don't store very well. This shouldn't be a problem, as they're quick and easy to prepare right before you need to use them.

This recipe is based on something I originally devised as a training tip for Neal's Yard Remedies Rose Facial Oil, when I worked for them several years ago. It involved mixing a teaspoon of oil with honey and pink clay to make a mask. The oils I chose are high in vitamins (camellia contains A, B, and C, and rosehip seed contains A and C) and antioxidants, and I would recommend using manuka honey.

Feel free to experiment with adding other ingredients to this mix, like mashed avocado or plain yogurt if you want a creamier texture.

Ingredients

2 teaspoons (10 ml) of honey (ideally manuka honey)
1 teaspoon (5 ml) of aloe vera
1 teaspoon (5 ml) of camellia oil

1 teaspoon (5 ml) of rosehip oil
½ teaspoon (2.5 ml) vitamin E
2 to 4 teaspoons (10 to 20 g) of pink clay or kaolin (white clay)

Equipment

small glass bowl or egg cup teaspoon

1 Measurewell. honey and aloe vera in the small bowl or egg cup and mix

2 Add camellia oil, rosehip oil and vitamin E, mixing thoroughly with ateaspoon.

3 Add the clay little by little until you reach the desired consistency.

USE

Spread on a freshly cleansed face and let sit for 10 to 20 minutes, preferably in a relaxing bath.

Apricot face scrub

This recipe is one that I have used for years to brighten up dull skin. I generally use almond oil because that's what I have on hand most often, but apricot and castor oils work great with honey to give a slightly thicker consistency. .

Make a small amount to use immediately as it doesn't keep well without preservatives and may separate due to lack of emulsifier. Using honey and ground rice in a recipe seems to provide an excellent growth medium for mold, and no matter how careful you are, there is a chance that during use, the water from your fingers will spill out. a path in the pot. I make a small amount and store it in a ½ fl oz (15 mL) jar of lip balm in the refrigerator. This means that I will be using it in a few days and that I don't need to use any preservative.

Ingredients

1 teaspoon (5 ml) apricot kernel oil

1   teaspoon (5 ml) castor oil

1 teaspoon (5 ml) of honey (manuka, if possible)

teaspoons (20 ml) of kaolin (white clay)

½ teaspoon of ground rice or rice bran a few drops of flower water 'orange tree, if necessary

small glass bowl or egg cup teaspoon
1 Measurer egg cup. apricot kernel oil, castor oil and honey in the small bowl

2 Add the kaolin and ground rice or rice bran, mixing everything well with a teaspoon.

3 If the mixture is too fine or you prefer a thicker texture, simply add more clay and stir until you get the desired consistency. If the mixture is too much thick, add a little orange blossom water to dilute it slightly. Store the leftover scrub in a small saucepan in the refrigerator and throw it away after a few days.

USE

Apply a small amount to damp skin and massage very gently (ground rice can be quite abrasive, so use light contact). If you find it too harsh or have sensitive skin, try ground almonds or jojoba pearls instead, which are available from many online suppliers that specialize in natural ingredients for making products. You can replace the kaolin with green or red clay, if you prefer. To remove the mask, rinse it off with lukewarm water and a washcloth. This scrub is also great to use on the body, if you must use it.

Along with cleansers, lip balms are on the list of products that you should never have to buy in a store again. They come in many forms and it is very easy to create professional looking products that would make great gifts as well. With the addition of some natural fruity flavors, they are a good way to engage kids in green living. In fact, many of the projects in this book are quite easy to do with children.

The balance of ingredients is much more flexible if you are going to put your balms in jars, as you can get by by being fairly mild. You can play around with different oils and butters to find a texture that you really like.

If you want to be more adventurous and use a twist-up stick, you'll have to stick to the ratio of oil and wax in the recipe quite strictly, as you need a much firmer consistency to make it. withstands use in the tube.

Soft butters

You can buy a lot of different soft butters online now, ranging from the most common shea butter to mango, apricot, olive and aloe butter. Of all these, shea butter is the thickest and creamiest and in my opinion makes the best lip balm. Cocoa butter is an essential ingredient as it adds firmness but melts instantly on contact with the skin. Beeswax not only keeps the whole formula together, but also helps it stay on your lips by forming a protective waxy layer.

Facial Cleansers

Honey, Milk, and Oatmeal Cleanser

<u>What you need:</u>

½ cup dry goat's milk, powdered

½ cup finely ground oatmeal

Medium bowl

Whisk

Clean, sterile jar with a lid

1 tablespoon honey powder (optional – you can also just add 2–3 drops of honey when you add the water)

Warm water

A clean rag

<u>How to make it:</u>

In a medium sized bowl, mix together the powdered goat's milk, ground oatmeal, and honey powder. Whisk the dry ingredients together well, making sure they are fully blended. Pour the mixture into a dry jar with a lid and store near your sink. To use the cleanser, put about ½ tablespoon of the dry mixture into the palm of your hand and add enough warm water to make a thin paste. (Adding the water at the time of use makes the cleanser shelf stable, whereas adding the water to the jar would cause the mixture to go bad quickly.) If you didn't use honey powder, this is when you would add a few drops of honey to the mixture in your hand.

Massage the cleanser over your face, using small circular motions to gently exfoliate and cover as much of your face as possible. Once you are satisfied, rinse off the cleanser with warm water and pat your face dry. This can be used daily to help mildly exfoliate, cleanse, and moisturize your face.

Aloe Refreshing Facial Cleanser

<u>What you need:</u>

5 tablespoons aloe vera gel (not liquid or oil)

3 teaspoons natural liquid castile soap

3 teaspoons jojoba, shea, coconut, or hemp oil

2–5 drops lavender essential oil

2 drops tea tree essential oil (optional)

¼ teaspoon honey

Sifter or fine mesh tea ball

1 teaspoon bentonite or kaolin clay

A clean plastic bottle or jar with a lid

Mixing bowl

Whisk

Funnel (if using a bottle)

<u>How to make it:</u>

Start by putting the aloe vera gel in the mixing bowl. Add the oils and honey and whisk together. Once the all the liquids are blended, add the castile soap and whisk gently, making sure not to get it too foamy with air bubbles. Sift the clay over the bowl and into the mixture and gently but thoroughly mix everything together so there are no lumps of clay. Cover the bowl and let it sit for about 30 minutes so that any air bubbles dissipate. Then use the whisk to stir the mixture just enough to make sure nothing settled. Pour the mixture into a jar or use a funnel to pour it into a bottle.

To use the aloe facial cleanser, dampen your entire face with warm water. Pour a nickel-sized amount of the cleanser into your dampened palms and rub your hands together to lather it. Apply the cleanser to your face, being careful not to get it into your eyes, and massage into the skin. Once you are finished lathering up your face, use warm water to rinse the mixture off and a dry, clean towel to pat the skin dry. This is safe for daily use and shelf-stable.

Face Scrubs

Gentle Face Scrub

<u>What you need:</u>

1 teaspoon baking soda

1 teaspoon finely ground oats

1 teaspoon honey

1 teaspoon coconut oil

Microwaveable bowl or measuring cup

Safety glasses

Oven mitt

Fork

Warm water

<u>How to make it:</u>

Put on your safety glasses. Place the coconut oil and honey into a microwaveable bowl or measuring cup and heat for 30 seconds. Remove the dish using an oven mitt and stir the mixture with a fork. Pour in the ground oats and baking soda and use the fork to mix the ingredients as well as you can.

To use this scrub, dampen your face with warm water. Scoop up a small amount of the scrub and massage in, using small circles, on your cheeks, nose, chin, jawline, and forehead. Rub well in areas where you are prone to oil build-up and acne. When you're finished, use a mild facial soap and warm water to wash off the scrub. Rinse your face with warm water and then pat dry with a clean towel. Use this scrub about once a week.

Basic Clay Facial Mask

<u>What you need:</u>

1 tablespoon bentonite clay

1–2 tablespoons distilled or rose water

1–3 drops tea tree, lavender, or chamomile essential oil (optional)

<u>How to make it:</u>

Pour 1 tablespoon of distilled water into a bowl or cup. Add a tablespoon of bentonite clay and stir. If the mixture is too thick (it should be the consistency of paste) add more water. Once the clay is mixed well with the water, add drops of essential oil, if desired. Mix the oils in well throughout the paste. This makes one face mask. Apply the paste over the face, being careful not to get it too close to your eyes. Allow it to dry then remove by washing your face gently with warm water. Pat dry. This mask is particularly beneficial for those with oily skin issues and acne problems.

Black Head Removal Peel

<u>What you need:</u>

1 tablespoon milk

1 tablespoon gelatin

Microwave-safe bowl or measuring cup

Spoon

Gloves

<u>How to make it:</u>

Pour the milk and gelatin into the microwaveable cup or bowl and stir together. Heat the mixture in the microwave for 5 seconds. Remove the dish, stir it well, put it back in the microwave and heat it again. Remove the dish and stir the mixture, making sure the gelatin has completely dissolved. If not, repeat the process until it has. Let it cool until it is safe to touch. Dip gloved fingers into the mixture and smear it on your nose, chin, cheeks, or forehead (wherever you would normally put a pore strip). Allow the peel to dry completely. Gently work up the sides and peel off the gelatin, being careful not to pull too fast. Afterward, use a facial cleanser and toner or moisturizer.

Cucumber Peel

<u>What you need:</u>

1 small cucumber or ½ of a large cucumber

½ cup hot water

2 green tea bags

¼ cup aloe vera gel (not liquid or oil)

1 tablespoon gelatin

A food processor or blender

Cheesecloth or fine strainer

Mixing bowl

Spoon

<u>How to make it:</u>

Before you begin, place the two tea bags in a cup of hot water to steep. Peel the cucumber and cut it into the smallest pieces you can. Put the pieces in a food processor or blender and pulse until puréed. Using a cheesecloth or fine mesh strainer, strain out the juice into the mixing bowl and dispose of the pulped meat. Remove the tea bags from the cup and stir in the gelatin. (Reheat the green tea if it is too cool to properly melt the gelatin.) Lay the tea bags flat and save them for later.

Add the aloe to the cucumber juice and stir well. Slowly pour in the green tea-and-gelatin mixture, stirring as you pour. Once you have mixed all of the ingredients together thoroughly, set the mixture to the side to cool for about 10–15 minutes. Once it has cooled, run the tea bags under the warmest water that is still comfortable to your skin. Press out all of the excess water. Use your fingers to apply the peel evenly over your face, keeping it out of your eyes. Lie back and place the tea bags on your eyes, making sure they are not dripping any excess water. Allow the mask to dry and the tea bags to cool. Remove the tea bags once they have cooled down. When the mask is dry, peel it off and rinse your face with warm water. Pat your skin dry with a clean towel.

Facial Toners and Astringents

Vinegar Toner for Sensitive Skin

<u>What you need:</u>

¼ cup apple cider vinegar

¾ cup distilled water, rose water or green tea

Clean jar or bottle with a lid

<u>How to make it:</u>

Mix all liquids together in a bottle. Shake well before every use, and then apply to a pad, cotton ball, or clean cloth and blot onto your face. Wait a few minutes before rinsing your face (if you want to: it isn't necessary to rinse) with cool water and patting dry. If you use green tea, store the toner in the refrigerator.

Vinegar Toner for Dry or Normal Skin Types

<u>What you need:</u>

⅓ cup apple cider vinegar

⅔ cup distilled water, rose water or green tea

5–10 drops tea tree oil

<u>How to make it:</u>

Mix the vinegar and water or tea together in a bottle. Add the drops of tea tree oil. Shake the bottle well before every use. To use, pour or dab the toner onto a pad, cotton ball, or clean cloth and blot onto your face. Wait a few minutes before rinsing your face (if you want to: it isn't necessary to rinse) with cool water and patting dry. If you use green tea, store the toner in the refrigerator.

Vinegar Toner for Oily Skin

What you need:

½ cup apple cider vinegar

½ cup distilled water, rose

water or green tea

5 drops tea tree oil

How to make it:

Mix the vinegar and water or tea together in a bottle. Add the drops of tea tree oil. Shake the bottle well before every use. To use, pour or dab the toner onto a pad, cotton ball, or clean cloth and blot onto your face. Wait a few minutes before rinsing your face (if you want to: it isn't necessary to rinse) with cool water and patting dry. If you use green tea, store the toner in the refrigerator.

Complexion Toner

What you need:

2 tablespoons honey

1 tablespoon lemon juice

½ cup rose water or witch hazel

A clean bottle with a lid

Funnel

Cotton balls

<u>How to make it:</u>

For the freshest lemon juice, squeeze your lemons right before you make your toner. To get the most juice from a lemon, zap it in the microwave for 15 seconds and then roll it around on the counter while applying slight pressure. This will help loosen up the pulp and let the juice flow more readily from the lemon.

In the bottle, pour the honey, lemon juice, and rose water or witch hazel (you may also use distilled water, if you wish). Put the lid on the bottle and shake well. To use this toner, pour a small amount on a cotton ball and coat your cheeks, chin, jaw, forehead, and nose with the toner. Be careful not to drip any into your eyes; if you do, quickly flush with eyewash or clean, distilled water. If you face feels tacky after it dries, use a damp cloth to gently wipe over the areas where you applied the toner, but don't scrub it.

Basic Witch Hazel Daily Astringent

<u>What you need:</u>

Witch hazel

5–10 drops tea tree oil

Distilled water (optional)

Clean and sterilized bottle with a lid

Pipette or dropper

Cotton ball or napkin or clean cloth

<u>How to make it:</u>

Take your empty bottle and fill it three quarters of the way full with witch hazel. Then use the pipette or dropper to add 5 drops of tea tree oil. Put the lid on the bottle, shake it up, and then apply a small amount to a cotton ball or napkin. Rub the astringent on your face. If the smell is too strong, or if you have sensitive skin, use a ratio of 2 parts witch hazel to 1 part water. If tea tree oil does not bother your skin or sense of smell, you can add a few more drops.

Use this astringent after removing makeup, before bed, and first thing in the morning to help your skin stay clean and clear

Face Moisturizers

Basic Facial Moisturizing Cream

<u>What you need:</u>

1 cup aloe vera gel (not liquid or oil)

¼ cup liquid oil (almond, jojoba, grape seed, hemp, etc.)

¼ cup coconut oil (can substitute palm or shea, but texture will be different)

¾ ounce beeswax (or ½ ounce carnauba, soy, or emulsion wax)

7–10 drops essential oil (lavender, chamomile, or other light florals are great)

5 drops vitamin E oil

A clean mixing bowl that can withstand heat

A stick blender

Double boiler or microwaveable bowl or measuring cup

Silicone spatula

Dropper

Kitchen scale

Safety glasses

Oven mitt

Clean and sterile jar with a lid, or a lotion bottle

<u>How to make it:</u>

This recipe can get a bit technical as you have to make an emulsion. That is, you have to combine an oil, a wax, and a water soluble liquid in a way to get them to come together and stay together. Once cooled, this should be a cream or lotion, but if it gets so hot as to melt the oils and waxes, it will no longer reform correctly.

Make sure all of your ingredients are ready to go before you start. Put on your safety glasses to protect your eyes, and make sure to use the oven mitt when handling the microwavable dishes or the double boiler. Measure out your wax and solid oil into either the top part of your double boiler or your microwave-safe dish. If you are using the double boiler, stir the ingredients occasionally as they melt. For the microwave, start with a 30-second blast, stir, and then continue with 15-second blasts until melted. Once your oils and waxes are completely melted, pour this into your mixing bowl using your oven mitts. Add in your liquid oil (almond, jojoba, hemp, etc.), stirring as you pour it in.

You should have your safety glasses on as you start the next part. Get your stick blender (or wand blender) and begin pouring in the aloe vera gel slowly as you blend on medium. Keep blending as solution whitens and begins to thicken. As it starts to become creamy, add in the essential oil and vitamin E oil. Keep blending the mixture for about ten minutes to make sure it has completely emulsified. Touch your finger to the lotion and smear it on your arm. If it is too greasy or oily, add more aloe vera gel while blending. If it is too watery, add more oil.

Once the mixture is completely blended, pour it into your jar and put the lid on. To use, put a small amount on your fingertips and massage it into your face. This solution can also work as a lotion.

Eye Compress for Dark Circles

<u>What you need:</u>

2 large reusable tea bags, or large empty tea bags, or thin, clean cotton squares

1 tablespoon chamomile tea (divided in half)

1 tablespoon green tea (divided in half)

2 teaspoons honey

1 large coffee cup or microwaveable cup

1 cup hot water
A spoon

<u>How to make it:</u>

Place ½ tablespoon of chamomile and ½ tablespoon of green tea in each tea bag. Seal or tie the bags shut. Mix the honey in the cup of hot water until it is dissolved. Drop the two tea bags into the hot water and use the spoon to make sure they are fully saturated. Allow them to steep for about 5 minutes. Pull out the tea bags and let them cool slightly, until they are warm to the touch. Lie back, place a tea bag over each closed eye, and relax for about 5–10 minutes. Remove the tea bags and rinse your face. Repeat the process a few times a week to help get rid of dark circles and bags under your eyes. The leftover honey, green tea, and chamomile tea is safe to drink, or you can use it as a toner for your face, but any excess should be disposed of or stored in the refrigerator.

Full Face Makeup

The biggest issue with homemade makeup is getting the perfect color, hue, and tone in your final product. Refer to the Colors section in Chapter 11 for a few starting points for different shades and colors. Always start with a very small quantity of any pigment or powder you are using and slowly add what you need to reach your desired shade. When you find your desired shade, then you can make a larger quantity. Because of the many options for coloration, the following recipes will have "pigmented powder" listed as an ingredient. This refers to the premade color powder you want to use for that specific makeup. When you make your colors, label them as "foundation #1" or "eye shadow #3" according to how many you have made, and make sure the recipe you used to make that specific powder is labeled the same.

To Make Loose Powdered Makeup Solid (Pressed Makeup)

<u>What you need:</u>

Loose, powdered makeup

Clean bowl

Fork or whisk

Rubbing alcohol

Empty makeup compact or shallow container with a lid

Clean spoon

Safety glasses

Dust mask

Gloves

<u>How to make it:</u>

Before you begin, put on the safety glasses, dust mask, and gloves. Start by pouring the loose powder into the bowl. Add a few drops of rubbing alcohol and then mix well with a fork or whisk. Try to press the makeup down. If it is still too crumbly, add a drop or two more alcohol. The makeup should be damp enough to stick together, but it will still be a little crumbly. Use the spoon to scoop up the mixture and put it into the compartment of a clean makeup compact or a shallow container. Use the spoon, your gloved fingers, or both to press the makeup firmly into the container. Make sure you apply the same pressure evenly all around. Once the makeup is flattened, you can spray a fine mist of alcohol over the top and use the back of the spoon to smooth it out, if you wish.

Allow the makeup to air dry. Once it is completely dry, the makeup will be solid and can be used like any store-brought brand. This can be done with any of the loose powdered recipes (eye shadow, foundation, bronzer, blush, highlighter, and finishing powder) in this book, as well as with old storebought makeup that has cracked or broken in the container. All you have to do is chip it all out, smash it up in a clean dish with a spoon, and then follow the same procedure as for your own powdered makeup.

Basic Loose Powder Foundation

<u>What you need:</u>

2 tablespoons zinc oxide (or arrowroot if you prefer not to use zinc; however, zinc has better coverage and sun protection)

1 tablespoon arrowroot powder

½ teaspoon clay (whichever suits your coloration best; make this 1 teaspoon if you don't use zinc)

1½ teaspoons pigmented powder that matches your tone; add more as needed

1 teaspoon translucent mica for oily skin

1 clean bowl or measuring cup

Measuring spoons

Whisk or fork

Sifter or fine mesh for sifting (metal, mesh tea balls work well)

Facemask and safety glasses

<u>How to make it:</u>

Before you begin, put on your safety glasses and facemask to prevent inhaling dust or getting the powder in your eyes. Sift the arrowroot powder and zinc (if using) into your bowl or cup.

This sifting will prevent clumping and help ensure your mixture is thoroughly combined. Then sift the clay into the bowl or cup and then whisk the powder. Finally, sift your premade pigmented powder into the mixture. Whisk everything together and make sure it is well combined and there are no clumps or powder sticking to the sides. Dip a clean makeup brush lightly into the powder, tap off the excess, and apply to the inside of your wrist to test out the color. Add more pigmented powder as needed if the color is not dark enough. If it is too dark, add more arrowroot powder. The last ingredient is translucent mica powder for oil absorption; if you choose, add it now and whisk everything together. Store the loose foundation in a container with a lid. The best containers to use are the ones made for loose powder makeup.

Bronzer

<u>What you need:</u>

⅛ teaspoon arrowroot powder

½ teaspoon cocoa powder

½ teaspoon cinnamon powder (not for everyday use) or

½ teaspoon rust red mica

⅛ teaspoon beetroot powder or pink mica

Pinch of gold or bronze mica powder

Whisk or fork

Sifter or tea ball made of fine mesh

Clean bowl or measuring cup

Dust mask

Safety glasses

Gloves Measuring bowls

<u>How to make it:</u>

Put on your safety glasses, gloves, and dust mask. (This isn't dangerous to the skin; the gloves are merely to keep from staining your hands or getting the powder on everything you touch.) Add each powder one by one, running it through a sifter or mesh tea ball if you have one, into your bowl or cup. This is only the base you are starting with. Use a whisk or fork to thoroughly blend the powders and make sure there are no lumps and the color is uniform. Now for the testing phase. Use your finger or a makeup brush and try the bronzer out on the top of your hand. See if the shade is what you are looking for. Use the cocoa powder to darken, the cinnamon or red mica to add more red, the pink mica or beetroot powder for cooler tones, and the gold mica for a warm glow (nutmeg can work for this, but it won't be as shimmery). Store the powder in a container with a lid and use for contouring or adding a summer glow to your cheek bones.

Highlighter

<u>What you need:</u>

¼ teaspoon arrowroot powder

¼ teaspoon white pearlescent mica

Small container with a lid

Mixing bowl or cup

A clean makeup brush

Safety glasses

Dust mask

<u>How to make it:</u>

Put on your safety glasses and dust mask before you begin mixing to prevent the dust from getting in your eyes or being inhaled. This recipe is rather simple, as the goal is to make a shimmery white powder to highlight parts of the face when contouring. The easiest way to blend the mixture is with a small makeup brush, though you can also use a small spoon. As with other powders, try it out and see if it is what you are looking for. If you want it to be more matte, add arrowroot powder, and for more shimmer, add more mica. Store in a small container with a lid.

Powder Blush

<u>What you need:</u>

¼ teaspoon arrowroot powder

Pinch of rose or kaolin clay

1 teaspoon pigmented powder pink hues: add more beetroot powder or pink mica

orange hues: add more annatto seed powder or orange mica

Bowl or cup

Sifter or fine mesh tea ball

Whisk or fork

Clean container with a lid

Safety glasses

Dust mask

<u>How to make it:</u>

Begin by putting on the safety glasses and dust mask for protection against the fine powders. Sift together the arrowroot powder, clay, and your pigmented powder. Use the whisk or fork to make sure it is all well blended. Test the powder out by dipping a clean brush into the finished product, tapping it on the side to remove excess, and then brushing onto your inner wrist for light complexions and the back of your hand for darker complexions. Add pigments, oxides, and powders to make the blush match the shade you were looking for. Even if you add only a pinch of powder, write it down so you can remember it later if you want to make more.

Finishing Powder or "Veil"

<u>What you need:</u>

¼ cup arrowroot powder

1 tablespoon cornstarch

1 teaspoon translucent mica

Large pinch of cocoa powder or your pigmented foundation powder (optional)

Sifter or fine mesh tea ball

Small mixing bowl

Whisk

Clean container with a lid

Dust mask

Safety glasses

<u>How to make it:</u>

Put on your safety glasses and dust mask before beginning to prevent the fine powder from being inhaled or getting into your eyes. Sift the arrowroot powder, cornstarch, and translucent mica into your mixing bowl. Whisk the powders together thoroughly. If you would like it to be tinted, add a pinch of cocoa powder or your pigmented foundation powder and whisk again. Pour the mixture into the container and seal with a lid. To use, dip your brush into the mixture and tap off the excess. Lightly brush the powder over your foundation and eye shadow to give your makeup an all-over smooth look.

Liquid Foundation

Concealer

<u>What you need:</u>

2 teaspoons jojoba, almond, olive, or hemp oil

1 teaspoon shea butter or coconut oil

⅓ teaspoon beeswax or ½ teaspoon soy or emulsifying wax

1 teaspoon witch hazel, rose water or distilled water

1 tablespoon aloe vera gel (not liquid or oil)

2 tablespoons zinc oxide

½ teaspoon of your pigmented foundation powder

Microwavable bowl or measuring cup, or a double boiler

Whisk or stick blender

Mixing bowl

Sifter or fine mesh tea ball

Dust mask

Safety glasses

Oven mitt
Small container lid

<u>How to make it:</u>

Put on your safety glasses before you begin. Place the shea butter or coconut oil and the wax into the top pot or bowl of your double boiler and melt it down. If using a microwave, place the shea butter or coconut oil and the wax into a microwaveable bowl or cup and heat for 30 seconds. Use your oven mitt to take it out and stir the mixture. Put it back in the microwave and blast for another 15 seconds, and then take out again, stir it, and check to see if it is melted. As soon as the mixture is completely melted, pour it into your mixing bowl. Whisk or use a stick blender on the mixture as you pour in the rest of the liquid ingredients (aloe vera gel, witch hazel or water, and liquid oil). Continue whisking or blending until the mixture becomes thicker and white throughout.

Put on your dust mask to avoid breathing in the fine powders. Sift in the zinc oxide and your pigmented foundation powder. Continue to blend the ingredients until they are well incorporated. Test a small spot on your face to see if the color matches what you are looking for. To darken, add cocoa powder in tiny amounts. To lighten, add clay powder or arrowroot powder in small amounts. Store the mixture in a container with a lid and use to mask discolorations and spots before you apply your foundation.

Basic Face Primer

<u>What you need:</u>

⅓ cup aloe vera gel (not liquid or oil)

½ teaspoon coconut oil

½ teaspoon vitamin E oil

Pinch of arrowroot powder, translucent mica or pigmented foundation powder

Small mixing bowl

Whisk

Microwavable dish or a double boiler

Clean and sterile container with a lid

Safety glasses

Oven mitt

<u>How to make it:</u>

Put on your safety glasses before you begin. In your microwaveable dish or the top pot or bowl of your double boiler, pour in the aloe gel and the coconut oil. Heat just until the coconut oil is completely melted. This should only take a minute or two in the double boiler. For the microwave, blast the mixture for 30 seconds. Whisk the ingredients, and if the coconut oil is still too thick, blast it for another 15 seconds. Once the coconut oil has melted enough to easily be whisked in with the aloe gel, pour the mixture into the mixing bowl. Add the vitamin E oil and whisk. Add a pinch of translucent mica or arrowroot powder (or your pigmented foundation powder, if you would like the primer tinted). Whisk the ingredients together until they are thoroughly mixed. Pour the solution into the container and put the lid on.

To use the primer, gently massage a small amount of the mixture over your face. The primer helps prevent oil build-up and prepares your skin for application of makeup for prolonged use. It also helps moisturize your skin and keep your face healthy by preventing drying of the face during makeup usage.

Simple Setting Spray

<u>What you need:</u>

¼ cup vegetable glycerin

¾ cup rose water

Clean bottle with a sprayer (sprayer should be able to "mist" liquid)

<u>How to make it:</u>

Pour the vegetable glycerin and rose water into the bottle. Put the lid on tightly and shake well. Setting spray is misted over your face once you are finished putting on makeup. When the light mist dries, your makeup will be more resistant to the wear and tear of the day.

Acne Prevention Setting Spray

<u>What you need:</u>

4 teaspoons vegetable glycerin

2 teaspoons witch hazel

¼ cup rose water or distilled water

3–5 drops tea tree oil

Funnel

Clean bottle with a sprayer (sprayer should be able to "mist" liquid)

<u>How to make it:</u>

Using a funnel, pour the glycerin, witch hazel, water, and tea tree oil into the bottle. Shake the solution well prior to each use. Spray a fine mist over your face once you have finished putting on your makeup to help seal it for the day. This solution is similar to the basic one, but is also beneficial for those prone to breakouts from using makeup, or just prone to them in general.

Cooling Setting Spray

<u>What you need:</u>

¼ cup aloe vera gel

¾ cup rose water or distilled water

3 drops vitamin E oil

Funnel

Clean bottle with a sprayer (sprayer should be able to "mist" liquid)

<u>How to make it:</u>

Use the funnel to pour the aloe vera gel and the rose water into the sprayer bottle. Add the drops of vitamin E and shake well prior to use. The aloe in this setting spray helps seal in your makeup and also refreshes and cools your face. This recipe is perfect for summer days and beating the heat.

Green Tea Setting Spray

<u>What you need:</u>

1 cup green tea

1 teaspoon honey

¼ cup rose water

3–5 drops vitamin E oil

Clean bottle with a sprayer (sprayer should be able to "mist" liquid)

Funnel

<u>How to make it:</u>

Start by making a cup of green tea. Add one teaspoon of honey and stir until it is dissolved. Let the cup of tea cool completely. Put the funnel into the bottle and pour in the honeyed green tea and rose water. Add the vitamin E oil and put in the sprayer. Shake well before every use. This solution lasts the longest when stored in the refrigerator as the green tea can sour over time, especially in warmer climates. Mist this finishing spray on your finished makeup to help give your face an antioxidant boost.

Body Care

Making soap can be a simple or extremely difficult process, and a complete explanation would fill a book all of its own. In this book, we will only cover a few simple recipes using what is called melt and pour soap. This is a soap pre-made with lye and vegetable glycerin, which is made from soy and palm oils. The difficult and dangerous aspects of cold process and hot process soap making have already been done. Melt and pour soap is available with added goat's milk, cocoa butter, shea butter, and even aloe. Not all brands are natural, so do your homework to make sure the kind you are purchasing is. The final product of melt and pour soap can be chopped up, melted down, and have ingredients added to it before it cools and becomes a useful bar of soap. (It can also be used in its base form, but it is odorless, has little minerals and nutrients, and can be drying. The recipes here will tell you how to take the melt and pour soap and add a few more natural ingredients to create a personalized bar. This lets you make your body clean without harsh chemicals and with all the healthy benefits you want added in. The soap comes with pre-lined marks. For the following recipes, cut along those marks to get the rough cubes required.

Soaps

Basic Moisturizing Soap

<u>What you need:</u>

8 cubes of melt and pour soap of your choice (or about 2½–3 cups)

1 tablespoon cocoa butter

1 tablespoon finely ground oatmeal

1 tablespoon powdered goat's milk

¼ tablespoon honey

5 drops vitamin E oil

5 drops almond extract

Double boiler or microwavable bowl or large measuring cup

Mixing bowl

Whisk

Loaf pan lined with wax paper, or a silicone soap, or candy mold or pan

Safety glasses Oven mitt

<u>How to make it:</u>

Begin by putting on your safety glasses. Put the chunks of soap, cocoa butter, honey, and oatmeal into the top of your double boiler or into the microwavable dish. Stir as it melts in the double boiler, or heat for 30 seconds in the microwave, remove it with the oven mitt, stir, and then continue to heat it in 15-second intervals while stirring in between until it is all melted. Add the powdered goat's milk as you whisk, making sure to break up any and all chunks. Then put in the drops of vitamin E oil and the almond oil. Whisk until everything is well blended, and then pour it into your prepared pan or mold and allow it to cool in a cool, dry place.

After the soap is completely cooled and hardened, take it out of the mold. If you used a pan, take it out, put it on a cutting board, and cut it into pieces suitable as individual bars of soap. Be aware that melt and pour soap can soften in hot and humid environments. Keep any extra soap in a cool, dry place, preferably wrapped in parchment paper, wax paper, or in a baggy. Use as a full body soap for smooth and moisturized skin.

Basic Bath Salts

<u>What you need:</u>

½ cup Dead Sea salt (or regular sea salt)

¼ cup Epsom salt (helps with muscle relaxation)

1 tablespoon baking soda

5–10 drops fragrance or essential oils
(optional)

Pigment (optional)

<u>How to make it:</u>

Blend the salts together with the baking soda in a large bowl. Once all the dry ingredients are fully integrated, add any dry colorant or pigment if you would like to color the bath. Stir and then add drops of fragrance or essential oils, spreading the drops around and not dripping them all in the same spot. Stir as you are putting the drops in, if you can. Continue stirring until all ingredients are well mixed. Store in a jar with a lid on it to prevent the product from getting damp.

When you take a bath, put 1–3 tablespoons of the salts in the warm water before you get in. Allow them to dissolve as much as possible so you don't have to sit on the gritty grains.

Body Scrub

Basic Sugar Scrub

What you need:

A clean and sterile jar with a lid

Granulated sugar

Oils of your choice (coconut, hemp, shea, jojoba, grape seed, etc.)

5 drops vitamin E oil

Chopstick or small dowel rod

How to make it:

Pour the granulated sugar into the jar, filling it three quarters of the way full. Then add your oils, putting enough in to cover the sugar. Use the chopstick or dowel rod to blend the mixture, making sure all of the sugar is coated with the oil. Once the mixture has settled, add more oil until it just covers the sugar, and then add the 5 drops of vitamin E oil.

To use the scrub, scoop a small amount out into your hand and massage into wet skin, making small circular motions. Once you have massaged it in well, wash your skin gently with soap and water, rinse, and then pat dry. Do not use this more than once a week. This scrub should leave your skin feeling very smooth and soft.

Body Moisturizer

Simple Lotion

<u>What you need:</u>

3 tablespoons coconut oil

1 tablespoon cocoa butter or shea butter

1 tablespoon beeswax or ¾ tablespoon soy wax

1 tablespoon aloe vera gel (not liquid or oil)

10 drops essential oil

3–5 drops vitamin E oil

Double boiler or microwavable bowl or measuring cup

Stick blender

Mixing bowl (if using a double boiler)

Bottle or container with a lid

Safety glasses

Oven mitt

<u>How to make it:</u>

Before you begin, put on the safety glasses. In the top of your double boiler, or in the microwavable dish you are using, place the wax, butters, and coconut oil. Melt in the double boiler or with a 30-second blast in the microwave. Stir, and if the microwave mixture is not melted, heat at 15second intervals, stirring in between, until everything has liquefied. Use your oven mitt to handle the hot dishes. If using a double boiler, pour the mixture into the mixing bowl. Use the stick blender to begin mixing the ingredients while slowly adding in the aloe vera gel. Keeping blending until the mixture has turned white and thickened. Add your essential oils and vitamin E oil to the mixture. Whisk everything to make sure it is all well incorporated. Pour into your container or use a funnel to put it in a lotion bottle. Use daily as a regular moisturizing lotion.

Hair Care

Hair Removal Sugar Wax

WARNING: Do not use this if you are not familiar with self-waxing. Be careful with the ingredients, as the initial wax is hot and must cool slightly. Use common sense and caution.

<u>What you need:</u>

2 tablespoons fresh lemon juice

2 tablespoons distilled water

1 cup sugar

Arrowroot powder or cornstarch

Large microwavable measuring cup

Spoon

Strips of clean and sterile cloth

Oven mitt

Safety glasses Clean, exfoliated legs

<u>How to make it:</u>

Don your safety glasses before you start. Pour the lemon juice and water into the measuring cup. Add in the sugar and stir. You can boil this lightly on the stove until it hits a light golden color. The wax will work better this way, but there's a greater risk of accidental burning. Heat at 30-second intervals, stirring in between, until the sugar is dissolved and the mixture begins to turn slightly golden. Once it is dissolved and mixed, pull it out and let it cool a bit. It may darken slightly. This is a good time to wash and exfoliate your legs. Pat them dry afterwards.

Lightly powder your legs with arrowroot powder or cornstarch, enough to make sure they are dry but not so much that a thick layer of powder remains.

Use a spoon or paintbrush to put thin layers of the mixture on your leg, brushing it downward, toward your feet. Do one strip at a time. Make the strip of wax and then lay a strip of clean cloth on top and pat it down onto the mixture. Pull the strip from the furthest end from your waist and rip backward against the hair growth. Repeat until all hair is removed. Rinse your legs and apply a moisturizer. Do not do this more than one a week.

Hair Conditioning Rinse

<u>What you need:</u>

1 cup apple cider vinegar

1 cup chamomile tea

A bottle or container you can take into the shower

<u>How to make it:</u>

Pour the apple cider vinegar and cooled chamomile tea into the container. Stir or shake well. After you have washed your hair in the shower, pour the mixture over your hair and massage it in. Let it sit for 5 minutes before rinsing your hair.

Natural Hair Lightener

<u>What you need:</u>

½ cup fresh lemon juice

½ cup chamomile tea

½ cup distilled water

A spray bottle

A towel

<u>How to make it:</u>

In the spray bottle, pour the lemon juice, cooled chamomile tea, and water.

Shake the bottle well. Put a towel over your shoulders and under your hair. Spray the mixture over your hair and massage it in. Spend 30 minutes to an hour in the sun, allowing your hair to dry. Afterward, rinse your hair out. Repeat as needed until your hair begins to lighten. This can take 3–5 times before you will see something like natural highlights. It will not work on all hair types and is not guaranteed on dyed hair.

Natural Hair Darkener

<u>What you need:</u>

1 cup very strong coffee

1 tablespoon cocoa powder

Measuring cup or shower safe cup

<u>How to make it:</u>

When you are in the shower, wash your hair as you normally would. Then coat your hair in the mixture and allow it to soak for 5–10 minutes. Rinse your hair thoroughly. Repeat as needed until your hair begins to darken. This will not work on all hair types and is not guaranteed on dyed hair. Be careful not to get the mixture into your eyes, as it may cause irritation. The darker the roast of the coffee and the finer the grind of the beans, the darker and stronger the coffee will be and the better it will be to darken your hair.

Conclusion:

here really are quite a few reasons to start making your own makeup, cosmetics, and beauty products. Time may be an issue for some, and the convenience of store-bought products is undeniable, but for the most part making your own is very much a "pro" rather than a "con." You may even enjoy it so much that you make a business out of it, and if nothing else, the joy of using something you made yourself, or giving it to someone you care about, is extremely satisfying. No one will know your product as well as you, and you will know everything that went into making your ideal cream, makeup, or facial mask. Not to mention, that makeup made with things like cocoa powder and cinnamon smells marvelous! Also, you will be saving money by making your own products, and you can adjust the quantities and frequency to meet your needs. With all these advantages, no wonder DIY makeup and beauty products is a no brainer!